Essential Oils

with the 12 Fundamental Essential Oils

Preface

ALEXANDRA LAVOISIER, PHARMACIST AROMATOLOGIST

Pharmacist dispensary, I present and recommend aromatherapy to my clients, daily. In recent years, essential oils have become trendy and a growing public shows interest in these natural products, without really knowing how to use them. May be discouraged by the number of existing essential oils and their broad therapeutic virtues, many people push the door of the pharmacy without knowing what might suit them. This guide is in this sense a great way to explore the aromatherapy and just get acquainted gradually with recipe creation to heal and create effective beauty products!

Essential oils offer a natural and effective alternative to traditional medicine and help reconnect with your body and learn to know better. The bias of this book - the one to propose effective recipes with only 12 essential oils - convinced me right away, because it addresses a major problem we face every day on the field: the trivialisation of aromatherapy. On the internet in beauty magazines or fashion, recipes on essential oils blooming everywhere without even informing readers about the basic principles of aromatherapy.

With this book, you can become an expert in aromatherapy and treat yourself safely. You will know the exact properties of each oil, its usage patterns and learn how to make your recipes with ease

owned by the owners themselves, not affiliated with this document.

Introduction

First of all, thank you for choosing this guide and let me tell you a little about the motivations that led me to write.

I was always conscious of the power of the plants to have been treated during childhood with unconventional medicine, including homeopathy and herbal medicine.

When I became interested in essential oils, I was quickly seduced. Nature gives the active ingredients, which when concentrated, have incredible power and replace chemistry. But then I was confused and almost discouraged. How to deal with more than 100 aromatic substances? Each new book I was reading, each new recipe I wanted to achieve, included the use of a new essential oil.

And how could I sort it out? How to treat minor injuries of everyday life without taking risks and without having to buy a new essential oil every time? And why not use these incredible oils for different functions?

I first made a real small pharmacy apothecary in order to make all the recipes that I found interesting. In the beginning, I created fairly complex mixtures including the use of many essential oils and vegetable oils. Then, little by little, I realized that the effectiveness of the oils was such that a few drops of essential oil were sufficient to transform a basic moisturizer into a powerful anti-wrinkle cream; and also when added to the shampoo for my hair or my mask, my hair was stronger and more shinny than ever!

But it's really in my travels abroad I realized that I always used the same essential oils, which thanks to their versatility allowed me to meet all my needs. It was during my first displacements and stresses that traveling induce that I finally learned the most about essential oils and their uses. And it's that experience that I wanted to share.

With this guide, you'll be able to look after your everyday aches and create beauty products and exceptional household maintenance products with only 12 essential oils. You will quickly be able to make quick, easy and cheap recipes for your own health as well as beauty recipes safely and without having to run out and buy a new ingredient in each recipe!

Welcome to the magical world of aromatherapy and enjoy the discovery!

Chapter 1

What is an Essential Oil?

An odorant

If essential oils are by definition "aromatic essences of plants", they should not be confused with those used in the field of perfumery where aromatic oils are called "perfume". These may be natural, but encounter increasingly synthetic flavors. Aromatic essences are also available in the kitchen, but as in the field of perfumery, the flavors are different than essential oils. It is to differentiate them from "flavors" as used in aromatherapy that they have been called "essential oils".

Therefore essential oil is a fragrant substance produced by certain plants.

Volatile substance that can be extracted in liquid form. Although called oils, these substances do not contain fat. A drop of essential oil deposited on a sheet of paper will evaporate without leaving any trace unlike oil.

A complex chemical composition

An essential oil can contain hundreds of molecules, each with very specific properties. They can be antiseptic, antibacterial, immunostimulant, etc. ... These molecules are grouped into "chemotypes" or biochemical families. This grouping done by scientists is based on their properties. It goes without saying that each essential oil can contain several chemotypes. For example: the essential oil of clary sage contains 250 different molecules: 75% of these molecules are part of the family of esters while 15% are from that of monoterpenols.

All these molecules work in synergy and allow the essential oils to be very versatile. Indeed, their fields of action are very broad the knowledge of chemotypes and their concentration in an essential oil determines what will be the benefits of this oil.

In the same plant, the effects of its essential oil, leaves or flowers taken in decoction may be different. Likewise, a plant may have multiple species, each containing different chemotypes from others. It depends on the place of harvest, climate or other crops grown nearby.

Essential oil chemotyped or craft?

Chemotyped essential oils come from laboratories that determine the exact biochemical structure of their products. These oils are usually combined in order to achieve a particular effect. Measurements are highly accurate, these essential oils are designed for well-defined medical treatments. These essential oils are preferred by scientists who want to standardize their production process. This process goes by planting, extracting and the composition of the oil itself.

Artisanal oils usually come from manual production not using sophisticated equipment. We then use native plants and even wild plants. These plants have the advantage of not having been treated and be completely natural. Supporters of the craft school say there is a slight difference between artisanal oils and chemotyped oils, but this difference does not affect their therapeutic properties. However, they argue that the crafted oils help fight better against local infections which may differ from one region to another.

Manufacturing Methods

There are several methods to extract the aromatic essence of plants and produce an essential oil. The extraction processes vary, in particular according to the intrinsic characteristics of the plant extract. Among these methods, distillation is the most common method, because the most reliable and economical.

The extractive distillation

This extraction method is known since the beginning of the use of essential oils and it is still the most commonly used today. In this method, water vapours pass,at low pressure, in a vessel where are placed the aromatic plants. The steam is then charged with fragrances contained in the plant, and then is sent to a refrigerated coil with cold water so that the steam condenses and becomes liquid. At the exit, the essential oil is separated with Floral Oil in a "essencier" by density difference.

Expression

This method, used only for agrumes, is to extract the essences pockets in the skin of citrus. then press the logs for the peels to release their essences. Note that for this method, the resulting product is not called essential oils, but simply "essence". This nuance in the name is explained by the fact that no biochemical change has occurred during the extraction process.

The effleurage

This process is used for plants, generally petals, that cannot stand the heat. The petals are immersed in a bath of animal fats that is heated repeatedly. Fat absorbs the essential oil contained in the plant. This is followed by the elimination of grease ointment to get only the essential oil. To do this, they use an alcohol solvent that absorbs the essential oil without the fat. Alcohol evaporates thereafter and there remains only the essential oil of high quality.

The by CO_2 Extraction

Modern mining method, yet it provides the essential oils of the highest quality. Vegetable masses are crossed by a stream of CO_2, thereby increasing the pressure and popping "naturally" bags of aromas. The essential oils obtained in this way have a biochemical constitution much closer to the original essence of the plant. This method, however, is uncommon, because very expensive.

Precautions and Recommendations for Practice

Aromatherapy is a very powerful medicine and molecules in essential oils may have contrary effects to the desired effects and / or negative when used in poor conditions. By following some simple basic rules you will be able to avoid these bad effects and enjoy the power of essential oils.

First, the use of essential oils is generally cons-indicated during the first 3 months of pregnancy for lactating women and young children. Past 3 months of pregnancy, some essential oils can be adapted, but subject to the advice of an aromatherapist.

Special precautions should be taken if you are asthmatic, epileptic, if you have a history of hypo or hyperthyroidism, hormone-related cancers or of stomach ulcer. If you are on medication, some essential oils can then be inappropriate.

In general, focus on external applications (friction massage) diluted in vegetable oil and consult your aromatherapist before taking an oral treatment or over a long period of time.

Never apply pure essential oil on the mucous membranes or near the eyes. In case of accident, rinse with a vegetable oil (olive oil) and water. Finally, follow the recommended doses: a drop is a drop, not two!

Also note that some essential oils are photosensitizing (including EO containing citrus molecules), so do not apply 6 hours before a sun exposure, as they can cause skin burns.

To keep them optimal, keep them in their original bottle that is slightly tinted to protect from UV rays and does not remove the condigoutte capsule. Also avoid exposing them to light. After use, close them as soon as possible, because essential oils are extremely volatile!

Finally, certain molecules contained in the essential oils can be irritating. If you have an allergy, ask your doctor and always perform a test inside of your elbow by mixing 1-2 drops of essential oil in a little vegetable oil, 48 hours before taking your treatment . If you notice redness, tingling, discomfort it simply means that this oil is not suitable for you!

How to use essential oils

Each essential oil has **unique properties** and therefore uses are also unique. There are 4 great potential ways to use essential oils: such as; oral, dermal atmospheric application, diffusion and use in a bath. Check the specifics of each essential oil in order to know its usage patterns.

Oral

As we have previously discussed, the essential oils **are irritating to the mucous membranes.** If ingesting (orally of course), it should be taken with a carrier such as honey, sugar, vegetable oil or a yogurt because they are not water soluble.

Some essential oils can be ingested in pure emergency and very small quantities. Always seek the advice of a specialist before taking an oral treatment.

Skin application

As for the ones taken orally, you must mix your essential oil with vegetable oil before applying it on your skin (with rare exceptions where you can apply the pure).

Vegetable oils therefore serve as support, but they also have properties on their own and complement and reinforce the action of essential oils. All vegetable oils can be used as support for essential oils and you do not have to buy them all.

Unlike an essential oil that is extracted from a plant or flower, a vegetable oil is extracted from the seed or a oleaginous fruit. It is obtained by pressure, cold or hot.

Below, you will find the vegetable oils that are widely used in aromatherapy and their main features and benefits:

🍃 Argan Oil

Origins from Morocco, argan oil comes from the fruit of the argan tree. Ideal to fight against drying of the skin Argan oil softens the skin. It also prevents skin aging by its firming and antioxidant action. Argan oil is also used to strengthen nails and revitalize dull, lifeless hair. It is also used in cooking and would be ideal for people with high blood pressure and cholesterol.

Attention many "fakes" of this oil exist, so always take those certified ECOCERT.

🍃 Arnica oily macerate

This oil is called macerate because it is obtained by macerating arnica flowers in neutral oil. The flowers release their active within weeks of maceration. The oily macerate arnica prevents the appearance of bruising and edema after a shock or a hit. Anti-inflammatory, it is also used to prevent muscle tension and aches and against joint and rheumatic pain. It is also very effective to relieve burns and sunburn. Used as massage oil after an intense physical effort, it is effective to relax your muscles and get fit!

🍃 Nuts Oil

Originally from Turkey, hazelnut oil is ideal for protecting and treating oily skin. It regulates sebum production effect, helps eliminate blackheads and tightens pores. It is very popular as "carrier oil" because it allows excellent penetration of the active present in essential oils without leaving a greasy film.

Jojoba Oil

From the deserts of South America, Jojoba oil, often renamed "desert gold" this oil is unique in its composition close to human sebum. Ally of your beauty, it penetrates easily into the skin without a trace of fat. Also effective on oily skin as very dry, it also prevents the appearance of wrinkles and helps firm the skin. Effective for oily hair, it also brings vitality, shine and flexibility to all hair types.

Macadamia Oil

Originally from Kenya, this oil is extremely rich in rare fatty acids. It is used to soften and protect sensitive, dry and mature skins. Extremely penetrating, it does not leave a greasy film that makes it ideal for massage. Lymphatic tonic, it is very effective against stretch marks. Applied to the hair, it protects against external aggressions.

St. John's Wort Oil

Herb St. John's wort is in many parts of the world. This oily macerate has anti-inflammatory, anti-trauma and healing. It calms and reduces burns consequences and also has psychic properties to fight against depression and anxiety states.

Calophylle Oil

From takamaka, a tree native to tropical regions of the Indian Ocean and Pacific, Calophylle oil has many powerful assets. Fluidity, it promotes blood circulation: it is therefore the preferred oil for all diseases related to circulation problems: varicose veins, hemorrhoids, rosacea. Antiseptic and anti-inflammatory, wound healing and it also protects from the sun.

🌿 Apricot Kernel Oil

From the apricot tree, this oil is known to improve skin tone because it is nourishing, moisturizing, regenerating and softening due to its high vitamin A, E and oleic acid. Recommended for dull skin, tired and devitalized to a real stunt. Combine with Jojoba oil for making a day care for the face!

🌿 Sweet Almond Oil

Native to Asia, it is now cultivated throughout the Mediterranean basin. Very versatile, it is the ally of the most delicate skin, like babies. Softening and toning, sweet almond oil is great to nourish the skin in depth and accelerate cell repair. Restorative, it helps fight against dry hair and gives a boost to your hair. Warning, this oil is allergenic for all sensitive to peanuts.

🌿 Aloe Vera Oil

From aloe, one of the oldest medicinal plants, aloe vera oil has exceptional nourishing and revitalizing properties. Renowned for its healing properties, it is also appreciated for its ability to regenerate the cellular system. Perfect for dry and mature skin it can be used in case of sunburn and nourish dry, brittle hair.

🌿 Avocado Oil

Rich in vitamins A, D and E, avocado oil is known for its moisturizing and regenerating properties. It is particularly suitable for dry and devitalized skin as it also softens, protects and strengthens. Excellent wrinkle is also a hair beautifying that resolves brittle and dry hair problems and stimulates regrowth.

Oil Carrot

The carrot oil encourages tanning and is also recommended as after-sun for the relaxation of the skin. Enhancer, it acts on the dull and tired skin by giving it a glow and delays the effects of aging.

I personally like to alternate vegetable oils that I use depending on my favorites of the season and my current needs. For example, I use a lot of argan oil and macadamia in winter when my skin is dry, and lighter oils such as jojoba oil in summer. To make my "health" recipes I still have an oily macerate arnica and a sweet almond oil or hazelnut of which are excellent carriers for dermal application. Finally, I buy the oils of carrot and apricot kernel when my skin needs a little bang in the winter!

Air use

Dissemination by olfactory pathway of essential oils allows perfuming the atmosphere to clean your home by destroying the virus and it is also used as insect repellent. Moreover, they also act against respiratory problems, stress and nervous conditions by acting directly on your psyche.

More or less noisy, effective or powerful, it is important to define your needs and peculiarities of your home before you make your choice.

There are 4 major families of broadcasters:

Diffuser by nebulization

This distribution method allows, through a powerful blast of air to separate the molecules of essential oils into very fine particles. This sophisticated technology allows to keep the exact benefits of each essential oil.

These broadcasters have far-reaching and can be used in very large areas up to 120sqm.

Ultrasonic diffuser or foggers

By emitting ultrasound, the diffuser allows the water and oil to be mixed to form a mist. Performed cold, this method has two advantages: it does not deteriorate the benefits of essential oils and is used to moisten the air. Furthermore, the distribution of the mist provides a nice visual effect.

These broadcasters have a more limited scope and can only be used for medium sized spaces (maximum 40sqm).

Ventilation diffuser

By blowing air on a blotter containing essential oils, the fan propels the microparticles of the essential oils into the air. This distribution method is fast and efficient, allowing to clean medium sized spaces (small room for example). Almost inaudible they are easily transportable and can accompany you in your car or at your desk.

Diffuser by soft heat

This diffusion technique is simple: under the effect of heat, aromatic particles are gradually propelled into the atmosphere. Very simple design, these broadcasters are generally very resistant, inexpensive and totally silent. However, they have a low reaching power (up to 20sqm).

In the bath

Add to bath water, essential oils have relaxing properties and can be beneficial in cases of fatigue, cooling or even viral disease. Essential oils are not soluble in water, you have to mix it before pouring in the bath. You can mix them with milk powder, liquid soap or vegetable oil. Never put more than 10 drops of essential oil in your bath.

How to choose my essential oils?

100% pure? 100% natural? Organic? With the success of essential oils, many brands are competing today on this very lucrative market. From one to another, quality differences can be significant, so it is important to know the selection criteria in order to take full advantage of the power of essential oils, safely. I recommend you always choose chemotyped oils (with the EOBBD or EOCT labelled), **100% pure and natural from organic agriculture.** In France, the oils from organic agriculture are certified by ECOCERT label.

- **100 % pure**: the essential oil comes from a botanical variety well-defined and clearly identified;

- **100 % natural**: the essential oil contains no substance other than that derived from the plant;

- **Label EOBBD** (Essential Oil Botanically and Biochemically Defined)

- **Label EOCT** (Essential Oil Chemotype)

From the packaging side, the essential oils must be contained in **opaque bottles**, and the following information must be indicated on the bottle: **the name of the plant** (plant species), its full scientific name (in Latin), **geographic origin**, **cultivation method** and the **method of obtaining the essential oil**. Also check the expiration date in order to know the maximum working time.

The price should not be a factor of choice in aromatherapy: Only high quality essential oils can pledge their efficiency!

If you can buy your essential oils in pharmacies, health food shops. Now those dedicated in particular to health and beauty products have especially expanded their range and excellent brands are sold there. So do not hesitate to ask until you find someone who could really answer your questions and point you in times of need. Note that not all pharmacists are specialized in Aromatherapy!

Finally, **always check the scientific name (in Latin)** before buying your essential oils. There are, for some essential oils, several varieties that may be similar. For example there are three types of essential oil of Eucalyptus: the radiata, the lemon and Globose that each have unique molecular properties. The scientific name allows you to purchase your essential oils in peace.

Chapter 2

My 12 Essential Oils

Heal with 12 essential oils, it is possible. The twelve essential oils that you'll find in this chapter are the most commonly used in aromatherapy, since their action spectrum is very broad. Used in synergy, these essential oils offer terribly effective solutions to cure your ills of everyday life and create your beauty elixirs.

Here are the twelve essential oils:

- **Exotic basil** (Ocimum basilicum)
- **Ho wood** (Cinnamomum camphora CT Linalol)
- **Noble Camomile** (Chamaemelum nobile)
- **Lemon Eucalyptus** (Eucalyptus citriodora)
- **Egyptian geranium** (Pelargonium X asperum)
- **Immortelle** (Helichrysum italicum ssp serotinum)
- **Laurel** (Laurus nobilis)
- **Spike lavender** (Lavandula spica)
- **Peppermint** (Mentha x piperita)
- **Ravintsara** (Cinnamomum camphora CT Cineole)
- **Tea tree** (Melaleuca alternifolia)
- **Ylang-Ylang** (Cananga odorata)

Glossary:
EO: Essential oil
VO: Vegetable oil
MO: macerate oily

Exotic Basil essential oil

Scientific name: Ocimum basilicum
Botanical family: Lamiaceae

Invigorating and vitalizing, essential oil of exotic basil is very effective for all digestive problems and stomach aches. Balancing the nervous system, it can boost its will and fight against stress!

Main Features :

- Antispasmodic
- Digestive
- Antiviral
- Antiseptic, anti-inflammatory
- Antibacterial
- Neuro-regulator
- Anti stress

Therapeutic properties:

Health

- Digestive problems (gas, bloating, upset transits, diarrheas, acidity).
- Spasmodic: intestinal cramps, menstrual pain, spasms, heartburn, vomiting, colic.
- Inflammatory pain: rheumatoid arthritis, rheumatism, muscle elongation.
- Migraines

Wellness
- Fatigue, depression, insomnia.
- Stress, Anxiety, Spasmophilia.

- Jet lag.
- Mental fatigue: overwork, lack of concentration, dynamism

Beauty
- Mature skin (antioxidant)
- Dull skin, tired and dull
- Acne-prone skin and / or fat

Precautions: Basil oil is very powerful. Do not use pure essential oil of exotic basil on the skin. Do not use over an extended period. Avoid the use orally. Not recommended for pregnant women, breastfeeding and for young children.

Basil exotic essential oil: Recipes

DIGESTIVE DISORDERS

In dermal application: 1 drop of EO Basil in 4 drops of vegetable oil on the abdomen after each meal.
Oral: 1 drop of pure Basil EO under the tongue or on a carrier, 3 times a day.

ARTHRITIS / CRAMPE / CONTRACTURE MUSCLE

In dermal application: 3 drops of EO in Basil 5 drops of vegetable oil arnica massage the painful area.

PAINFUL PERIODS

In dermal application: 2 drops of basil exotic EO in 4 drops of vegetable almond oil massage in the lower abdomen, several times a day.

HEARTBURN

- EO Basil 2 drops
- EO Camomile 2 drops
- EO Peppermint: 1 drop

Use: Take 2 drops of the mixture on a piece of sugar or a teaspoon of honey before meals and massage in with 3 drops of the mixture on the solar plexus after every meal.

FATIGUE (dermal application or olfaction)

By dermal application: 3 drops of essential oil in a vegetable oil, 5 drops on the belly several times per day.

Air diffusion: Mix 2 drops of essential oil of exotic basil 1 drop of EO Ylang Ylang in your diffuser, 2 times a day.

STRESS

In dermal application: Mix 4 drops of basil EO half a teaspoon of vegetable oil and apply the mixture to massage the solar plexus, neck, spine and stomach.

DULL SKIN WITHOUT GLOW

- EO Basil: 30 drops
- Organic grapefruit Hydrolat: 100 ml

Use: Add 30 drops of essential oil in your grapefruit hydrolat and apply morning and evening.

Ho wood Essential oil

**Scientific name: Cinnamomum camphora CT
Linalol
Botanical family: Lamiaceae**

Originally from China, essential oil Ho wood offers an alternative choice to the Rose wood oil. Excellent anti-infectives, its regenerating and purifying properties make it an ideal ally against aging and skin problems.
Main Features:

- Immune stimulant
- Antiviral
- Antifungal
- Pest control
- Analgesic
- Regenerative tissue

Therapeutic properties:

Health

- ENT infection: bronchitis, influenza, nasopharyngitis
- Urinary and gynecological infections: cystitis, vaginitis, vaginal discharge, vulvite
- Skin or gynecological fungal infections

Wellness
- Depression
- Nervous exhaustion, overwork

Beauty
- Acne, eczema (dry or superinfected)
- Mature skin, wrinkled

Precautions: Use preferably diluted to 20% in vegetable oil for skin applications. You can use,exceptionally, pure to disinfect open wounds. Do not use for pregnant or lactating women. Do not use over an extended period. Not recommended for young children. Avoid the use orally.

Essential oil Ho wood: Recipes

URINARY INFECTIONS AND GYNAECOLOGICAL

- EO Ho wood: 3 drops
- VO Hazel: 2 drops

Use: Apply 4 drops of the mixture in local application on the lower abdomen.

SKIN DISORDERS
- EO Ho Wood: 2 drops
- VO jojoba: 2 drops

Use: Apply 4 drops of the mixture under the concerned areas.

ACNE
- EO Ho wood: 10 drops
- EO Niaouli: 10 drops
- EO Tea tree: 10 drops
- VO Jojoba: 30 ml

Use: Apply 2 drops of the topical mixture several times a day on clean skin until disappearance.

FACIAL ANTI-WRINKLE

- EO Ho wood: 1 drop

Use: Mix 1 drop of essential oil to a daily dose of day cream (or night), it prevents the appearance of wrinkles and stimulates the regeneration of skin tissue.

REPULPANT MASK

- Cocoa butter: 10 ml
- Vegetable argan oil: 10 ml
- Vegetable apricot oil: 10 ml
- Shea butter: 20 ml
- EO wood Ho: 15 drops

Use: Mix all ingredients and put them in an airtight jar clean. Apply evenly to the face and neck for 15 minutes, 1-2 times a week.

ENT DISORDERS (bronchitis, influenza, nasopharyngitis)

- VO almond: 15 ml
- EO Ho Wood: 5 drops
- EO Niaouli: 5 drops
- EO Ravintsara: 5 drops

Use: Apply a few drops of the mixture in massage on the solar plexus and along the spine.

Noble Camomile essential oil

Scientific name: Chamaemelum nobile
Botanical family: Asteraceae

Calming the central nervous system, it is, by far, the best anti-stress essential oil. It is also popular to relieve skin problems and digestive disorders. Very soft, it can be used by the whole family!

Main Features :

- Antispasmodic
- Anti-inflammatory
- Hypo-allergenic
- Healing
- Digestive tonic
- Softening

Therapeutic properties:

Health

- Spasmodic disorders: bloating, flatulence, painful periods
- Nervous asthma
- Pruritic dermatological and / or allergic
- Rheumatism, muscle tensions
- Pental pain, migraine
- Mild sedative (child friendly)

Beauty
- Eczema, psoriasis, acne, herpes zoster, dermatitis
- Sensitive, irritated skin
- Razor fire

Wellness
- Agitation, anxiety, anxiety, stress
- Shock or emotional trauma
- Sleep disorder

Precautions: Very good tolerance: This is one of the few essential oils to be used for children. Suitable for pregnant women. Do not use pure on the skin.

The essential oil of noble camomile: Recipes

SEXUAL FEMALE FATIGUE

- EO noble Camomile 2 drops
- EO Ylang-ylang 2 drops
- EO Ho wood: 1 drop
- VO apricot kernel 10 drops

Use: Apply 4 drops of the mixture in the bottom of the vertebral column, 2 times daily for 1 week.

TENSED NECK, TORTICOLLIS (in adults)

- EO noble camomile: 5 drops
- EO Ravintsara: 15 drops
- EO Lemon Eucalyptus: 10 drops
- MO arnica: 20 drops

Use: A few drops of gentle massage and energetic mixture on your back and neck muscles.

SENSITIVE SKIN, ROSACEA

Mix 1 drop of essential oils in your dose of face cream every morning.

EMOTIONAL SHOCK

In dermal application: 3 drops on the solar plexus
Oral: 1 pure drop of noble camomile under the tongue

ANTISTRESS (in olfaction, then massage)

Start by taking a few minutes to inhale the essential oil to calm and mix 4 drops of EO to a VO nuts of your choice and gently massage your solar plexus, your stomach and your neck. Apply 2 times a day until calm returns.

ANXIETY

- EO noble Camomile 3 drops
- EO lavender: 10 drops
- VO Sweet Almond: 15 ml

Use: Apply 1 to 2 drops plexus massage + arch at night

SKIN IRRITANT SENSITIVE (oil massage)
- EO noble camomile: 10 drops
- MO Wort: 30 drops

Use: Apply the mixture on the affected areas until improvement.

Lemon Eucalyptus Essential Oil
Scientific name: Eucalyptus citriodora
Botanical family: Myrtaceae

Anti-inflammatory and anti-pain, this essential oil has extraordinary joint and muscular benefits. Stimulating the immune system, it allows notably to face the winter infections and drive away mosquitoes in the summer.

Main Features :

- Anti-inflammatory (articular, muscular)
- Analgesic
- Insectifuge
- Genital and urinary anti-inflammatory
- Antispasmodic
- Skin soothing
- Stimulating blood circulation

Therapeutic properties:

Health
- Joint and muscle pain (aches, stiff neck, pulled muscle)
- Joint inflammation (inflammatory arthritis, rheumatoid arthritis, rheumatism)
- Prevention of winter infections (flu, cold, cough)
- Inflammations urogenital: cystitis, vaginitis, vaginal discharge

Beauty
- Skin irritation (mycosis, tinea) itching
- Infected acne
- Cellulite

Wellness
- General fatigue
- Light insomnia
- Stress, sadness

Precautions: May be irritating to sensitive or irritated skin: Always dilute your essential oil with vegetable oil and made an awareness test before applying. Do not use in children under 8 years old. Do not use in pregnant women under 3 months or lactating.

Oil of Lemon Eucalyptus: Recipes

PAIN, JOINT INFLAMMATION

- EO Lemon Eucalyptus: 3 drops
- EO Everlasting: 1 drop
- VO: 10 drops

Use: Apply the mixture gently massage in painful areas.

CYSTITIS, VAGINITIS

- EO Lemon Eucalyptus 2 drops
- VO: 5 drops

Use: Apply the mixture on the lower abdomen and massage.

SHINGLES

- EO Ravintsara: 1 drop
- EO Peppermint: 1 drop
- EO exotic Basil 1 drop
- EO Lemon Eucalyptus 1 drop
- MO: 4 drops

Use: 2 to 4 drops of the mixture on the belly button or the painful area 8 times a day until symptoms disappear.

INSECT BITES (repellent and curative)

- EO citronella java: 1 ml
- EO Lemon Eucalyptus: 2 ml
- VO: 10 ml

-Repellent: Apply topically on the exposed members from 10 to 12 drops of the mixture 4 to 5 times per day.
-Curative: Apply 1 to 2 drops on the bite.

NOSE MOUTH (In diffusion in air)

- EO Eucalyptus
- EO Ravintsara
- EO Niaouli
- EO Lavender true.

Use: Spread the mixture into your diffuser 1 hour before bedtime.

SINUSITIS
- EO Eucalyptus 1 drop
- Hazelnut oil: 4 drops

Use: Apply the mixture to 4 times daily on the front in times of crisis.

Egyptian Geranium Essential Oil

Scientific name: Pelargonium X asperum

Botanical family: Geraniaceae

Anti-infective and antifungal, Geranium essential oil from Egypt is very effective for beauty treatments and to treat skin diseases such as fungal infections or eczema, hair care and slimming treatments.

Main Features :

- Antibacterial
- Antifungal
- Hemostatic and healing
- Skin astringent tonic
- Analgesic and anti-inflammatory
- Mosquito repellent

Therapeutic properties:

Health
- Skin and gynecological fungal infections
- Wounds, cuts, burns
- Epistaxis (nose bleeds)
- Hemorrhoids, phlebitis
- Osteo-articular rheumatism

Wellness
- Stress
- Deep asthenia
- Anxiety

Beauty
- Oily skin, acne
- Eczema, psoriasis, shingles, impetigo

- Thinning
- Stretch marks (prevention)

Caution: No special against-indications, except it is not recommended for pregnant and lactating women.

Geranium essential oil of Egype: Recipes

LIFTING CREAM

- VO jojoba: 30 ml
- EO immortal: 6 drops
- EO geranium 3 drops
- EO wood Ho: 3 drops

Use: Mix the ingredients in a bottle sealed pump and apply every morning on face and neck.

MASK SKIN wrinkled

- VO Lawyer: 1 teaspoon
- Pink clay: 3 tablespoons
- EO Geranium: 1 drop

Use: Apply to the skin in thin layers. Let stand 15 minutes then rinse.

DERMATOSES (psoriasis, eczema, hives)

Use: Apply 3 drops in a vegetable oil.

TONIC OIL

- EO Geranium: 5ml
- VO Sweet Almond 100 ml

Use: Apply the mixture on the body, massage for a tonic effect.

EPISTAXIS (nose bleeds)

Use: Put 1 drop on a cotton swab in the nose to stop bleeding.

PTOSIS (falling Breast)

- EO Geranium 2 drops
- Vera cream aloe gel

Use: Apply 1 time a day on the breasts to firm. For maximum effect, keep your aloe vera gel in your refrigerator.

HEMORRHOIDS

- EO Geranium 2 drops
- VO Hazel: 2 drops

Use: Apply 2 times a day until improvement of hemorrhoids.

ACNE

Use: Put 1 drop of EO on a cotton swab and apply the pimples 2 times a day on clean skin.

Immortelle Essential Oil

Scientific name: Helichrysum italicum
Botanical classification: Asteraceae

This essential oil is perfect for small traumatic everyday ailments: Bumps, bruises, wounds. It is also the ally of mature skin by its firming tissue and healing action.

Main Features :

- Anti-hematoma
- Anti-phlebitis
- Lymphotonic
- Anti-inflammatory
- Healing

Therapeutic properties:

Health

- Hematomas (bruises) external and internal blows, bumps, sores, burns
- Phlebitis, varicose veins, blood circulation problems
- Joint pain: arthritis, arthritis, rheumatism
- Spider veins, erythrose (diffuse redness of the skin), cyanosis
- Bronchitis, cough

Beauty
- Deep wrinkles, fine lines
- Rosacea
- Scars, stretch marks,
- Eczema, psoriasis
- Acne, acne scar

Wellness
- Psychological injury and trauma,
- Physical abuse and / or psychological,
- Loss of confidence

Precautions: The immortal EO is very powerful. Do not use in pregnant women, nursing as well as young children. Not recommended for people with allergies or epilepsy.

Immortelle essential oil

SCAR

- EO Immortelle: 3 drops
- VO Rosehip: 2 drops
- VO Calophylle: 2 drops

Use: Massage your scar with this mixture two times a day until improvement.

CONTUSION, BRUISING, HEMATOMA

- EO Immortelle: 2 drops
- VO Arnica: 2 drops

Use: Apply to the affected area 3 times a day for 24 hours.

VARICE

- EO Immortelle: 2 drops
- VO Calophylle: 2 drops

Use: Massage your varicose vein with this mixture two times a day.

TOOTH ABSCESS

- EO Immortelle: 1 drop
- EO Basil Exotic: 1 drop
- EO Laurel: 2 drops
- EO Peppermint: 1 drop
- VO Wort: 4 drops

Use: Apply the mixture to the gum 3 times daily for 1 to 2 days.

PREVENTION OF STRETCH MARKS

- EO Geranium of Egypt: 1 drop
- EO Immortelle: 1 drop
- EO Ho wood: 1 drop
- VO argan: 70 drops

Use: Apply 10 drops of the mixture in the morning and evening on the belly, thighs and breasts, 6 days a week from the 4th month of pregnancy.

RIDES

- EO Immortelle: 4 drops
- EO Roman Camomile 2 drops
- VO Jojoba: 10 ml
- VO Argan: 20 ml

Use: Apply a dab of the mixture on your face, neck and in between breasts in the morning and evening by gently massaging until completely absorbed.

Bay Laurel Essential Oil

Scientific name: Laurus nobilis

Botanical family: Lauraceae

This versatile essential oil has cleansing, purifying and soothing benefits. This essential oil works miracles for facials and teeth. It relieves joint pain and brings confidence and strength psychologically.

Main Features :

- Antiviral
- Fungicide
- Infection
- Antibacterial
- Analgesic
- Antispasmodic
- Anti-inflammatory
- Anticoagulant
- Regulating the nervous system

Therapeutic properties:

Health

- Infections and inflammation in the mouth (Mouth ulcers, gingivitis)
- Skin infections (Pressure sores, boils, abscesses)
viral diseases (flu, cough)
- Chronic respiratory diseases (bronchitis, asthma, chronic sinusitis)
- Indigestion, flatulence
- Neuralgia

Beauty
- Scar, bedsores

- Wrinkles and fine lines (prevention and care)
- Oily skin, acne
- Hair loss, hair soft, dull

Wellness
- Anxiety, depressive disorders
- Lack of self-confidence, fear of public speaking
- Memory loss

Caution: Possible skin reaction. Do not use pure on the skin. Do not use in pregnant women, nursing or young children. Use low-dose only.

Oil of Laurel: Recipes

BRONCHITIS, SINUSITIS CHRONICLES

Use: Put 3 drops of noble Laurel EO in a bowl of hot water and inhale the mixture for 10 to 15 minutes several times a day.

APHTHAE (local application)

Use: 1 pure drop on aphthae, 2 times a day until disappearance.

NERVOUS (before an exam or speaking in public)

- EO noble Laurel: 1 drop
- EO Peppermint: 1 drop

Use: Take the 2 essential oils on a support (teaspoon of honey or sugar) in oral and apply 1 undiluted drop on the inside of each wrist and breathe deeply.

MYCOSES

In dermal application: 2 pure drops on the fungus, morning and night for 3 weeks. Make a break for a week and start again until it disappears.

PRESSURE ULCER

- EO Laurel: 2 drops
- EO Spike lavender 3 drops
- VO Wort: 20 drops

Use: Apply the mixture on the wound three times a day until improvement.

HAIR (activate the shoot / tone the scalp)

Use: Mix 2 drops of essential oil of Laurel to your usual shampoo dose.

ACNE PURULANTE

- EO Laurel: 5 drops
- EO Spike Lavender: 5 drops
- EO Tea tree: 5 drops
- VO Macadamia: 5 ml

Use: Apply a few drops of the mixture on the affected areas 3-4 times a day until improvement.

PARODONTITIS, GINGIVITIS

- EO noble Laurel: 1 drop
- EO Tea tree: 1 drop
- VO Wort: 2 drops

Use: Massage your gums with this mixture several times a day until improvement.

Spike Lavender Essential Oil
Scientific name: Lavandula spica
Botanical family: Lamiaceae

Valued for its healing properties it is very effective on wounds and fungal infections. Soothing, it is also used to relieve insect bites and burns.

Main Features :
- Antitoxic
- Fungicide
- Antiviral and immune stimulant
- Healing
- Analgesic, analgesic
- General tonic

Therapeutic properties:

Health
- Headaches, migraines
- Burns, sunburn
- Skin and gynecological fungal infections
- Bronchitis, laryngitis, sinusitis, otitis, rhinitis
- Cramps, contractures
- Rheumatism
- Insect bites, wasps, jellyfish, scorpions

Beauty
- Dermatoses: herpes labialis, eczema, chickenpox, Zona, rosacea, psoriasis ...
- Crevices, cracks, damaged by the cold lips

Wellness
- Asthenia nervous depression

- Nervous fatigue, physical
- Stress, overwork
- Irritability, mood swings
- Anxiety and emotionality

Precautions: No restrictions except for pregnant women, breastfeeding and children under 7 years.

Oil of Spike Lavender: Recipes

SINUSITIS

- EO Peppermint 3 drops
- EO Spike Lavender: 2 drops
- EO Tea tree: 4 drops
- EO Eucalyptus dives: 1 drop

Use: 3 drops 3 times a day on the front and on a tissue to inhale at will.

SUNBURN

- EO Spike Lavender: 2 drops
- Aloe vera gel 2 drops

Use: After a sunburn, apply the mixture 2-3 times a day until improvement (For immediate relief, keep the aloe vera gel in the fridge!)

SKIN BURNS, ABRASIONS

- EO Spike Lavender: 60 drops
- EO Ho wood: 20 drops
- EO Laurel: 10 drops
- EO Wort: 10 drops

Use: Place first the burn under cold water for at least 5 minutes then remove. Then apply 8 drops of the mixture on the wound 6 times a day.

BITE WASP, SCORPION, MEDUSA, SNAKE BITE

- EO Spike Lavender 3 drops

- EO Immortelle: 1 drop
- EO Lemon Eucalyptus 1 drop

Use: Apply the mixture on the pure area (every 5 min for half an hour and then 3 to 4 times daily for one or two days)

SLEEP DISORDER, ANXIETY

Use: Put a pure spike lavender EO drop on your pillow before bedtime.

CHAPPING, LIPS ABIMEES

- EO Spike Lavender: 1 drop
- VO Wort: 5 drops

Use: Apply the mixture on the affected areas three times a day.

Peppermint Essential Oil
Latin name: Mentha piperita
Botanical family: Lamiaceae

Very versatile, essential oil helps heal many ailments of daily life: migraines, digestive problems, nausea and hangovers.
Main Features :

- Analgesic
- Antispasmodic
- Stimulating digestive and pancreatic
- Regulatory and liver protective
- Anti-inflammatory
- Stimulating the nervous system

Therapeutic properties:

Health

- Headache, Migraine
- Rhinitis, sinusitis, otitis
- Nausea, vomiting
- Acute diarrhea
- Motion sickness, vertigo
- Neuralgia, sciatica, arthritis, rheumatism, tendonitis
- Cystitis, colitis
- Hypotension

Wellness
- Shock, trauma
- Asthenia physical, mental and sexual
- Trac, Anxiety

Beauty
- Sweat
- Skin problems (eczema, allergic skin reaction)
- Foul breath

Precautions: formal ban for pregnant and lactating women and infants under 30 months.

Oil of Peppermint: Recipes

NAUSEA (SICKNESS)

- EO Peppermint: 10 drops
- EO Basil: 10 drops
- EO Lemon: 10 drops
- EO Apricot kernel: 8 ml

Use: Apply the mixture on your chest when you experience nausea in transport.

TENNIS ELBOW, TENDONITIS, RIP MUSCLE

- EO Peppermint: 20 drops
- EO Lemon Eucalyptus: 20 drops
- EO Immortelle: 30 drops
- EO exotic Basil: 10 drops
- MO arnica: 20 drops

Use: Apply the mixture locally 5 times a day for 5 to 7 days.

CONTUSIONS, ELONGATION MUSCLE TOOTH EXTRACTION

- EO Immortelle: 3 drops
- EO Noble Laurel; 1 drop
- EO Peppermint: 1 drop
- VO Callophyla: 5 drops

Use: Apply the mixture every hour for 24 hours.

CELLULITE (with obesity)

- EO Peppermint: 20 drops

- EO Lemon Eucalyptus: 10 drops
- EO Immortelle: 10 drops
- VO apricot kernels: 60 drops

Use: Apply morning and evening, massaging until completely absorbed

HANGOVER

- **Oral way:** 1 pure drop under the tongue
- **Cutaneous way:** 1 pure drop on temples to massage. Apply several times a day.

FETID BREATH

- **Oral way:** 1 drop on your toothpaste

LUMBAGO

- EO noble Laurel: 1 drop
- EO Peppermint: 1 drop
- EO Lemon Eucalyptus 2 drops

Use: Apply the mixture on the affected area, 5 times a day until improvement.

Ravintsara Essential Oil

Scientific name: Cinnamomum camphora CT Cineole

Botanical family: Lauraceae

Aromatherapy pillar of the diversity of its applications, essential oil Ravintsara is indicated for all ENT infections. Antiviral and stimulating the immune system, it is used for many infections and is suitable for the whole family! In Malagasy it is called "good leaf for all!"

Main Features :

- Antiviral
- Anti-inflammatory, analgesic
- Antiseptic, antiviral
- Antispasmodic
- Muscle relaxant

Therapeutic properties:

Health

- Rheumatic pain, joint pain
- Headaches, migraines
- Canker sores, cold sores
- Flu and viral infections
- Fatigue, stress, nervousness
- Chronic allergies
- Colds

Wellness
- Insomnia
- Depression

- Anxiety, nervous exhaustion

Beauty
- Acne, skin infections

Precautions: No special instructions for this essential oil also well suited for children and adults. Not recommended during the first 3 months of pregnancy.

Oil of Ravintsara: Recipes

BEGINNING OF FLU:

- EO Ravintsara: 3 drops
- VO macadamia: 3 drops

Use: Apply the mixture by rubbing on the neck, chest and wrists 3 times a day

TENSION NECK

- EO Peppermint 2 drops
- EO lemon eucalyptus: 4 drops
- EO Ravintsara: 2 drops
- VO Macadamia: 10 ml oil

Use: Apply the mixture and massage your neck 1-2 times a day for 4 days.

HAIR LOSS

- EO noble Camomile 15 drops
- EO Immortelle: 15 drops
- EO Ravintsara: 70 drops

Use: Mix 2 drops of the mixture in your usual shampoo dose.

MEMORY LOSS

- 20 drops Ravintsara
- 20 drops Peppermint
- 10 drops of Basil
- 50 drops of Apricot kernel

Use: Apply 4-6 drops of the mixture on the solar plexus, 3 drops on the wrists and 2 drops in the center of the forehead, 2 times a day.

BUTTON FEVER IN ADULTS

- EO Ravintsara: 20 drops
- EO Peppermint: 20 drops
- EO Spike lavender: 10 drops
- VO Apricot kernel: 50 drops

Use: Apply 2-3 drops of the mixture 8 to 10 times daily for 2 or 3 days (intervene at the first symptoms: redness, swelling, itching)

FEVER

Add 3 drops of essential oil Ravintsara and 3 drops of essential oil of Niaouli to a tablespoon of vegetable oil to your bath water.

Tea-Tree Essential Oil
Scientific name: Melaleuca alternifolia
Botanical family: Myrtaceae

Stimulating the immune system, it is also a powerful antiseptic that cleanses and invigorates the scalp and skin.
Main Features :

- Bactericidal broad spectrum
- Antifungal
- Antiviral
- Aest control
- Anti-inflammatory
- Purifying, it sanitizes problem skin
- Purifies, cleanses and tones the Scalp
- Stimulating and tonic
- Positivist

Therapeutic properties:

Health
- Oral infections: ulcers, abscesses, gingivitis
- ENT. infections Ear infections, sinusitis, pharyngitis, nasopharyngitis
- Gynecological infections: hemorrhoids, vaginitis, pelvic inflammatory disease
- Urinary tract infections: cystitis, urethritis

Beauty
- Skin problems, acne
- Localized infections
- Oral Care
- Antiseptic gels

- Purifying soap
- Personal hygiene

Wellness
- Physical and nervous exhaustion
- Chilliness

Precautions: Forbidden in pregnant women, breastfeeding and children under 10 years. For use on short period (maximum 5-6 days for infectious problems).

Oil of Tee Tree: Recipes

ACNE

- EO spike lavender 2 drops
- EO Tea Tree: 2 drops
- EO Peppermint: 1 drop
- VO hazelnut: 5ml

Use: Apply morning and evening mixture on each point.

TEETH WHITENING

- EO noble Laurel: 10 drops
- EO Tea Tree: 40 drops
- EO Peppermint. 30 drops
- VO Wort: 20 drops

Use: 2 drops on toothpaste treatment of dental stash + halitosis / dental calculus

OTITIS (Viral or bacterial infections, air conditioning, air, altitude)
- EO Ravinstara: 30 drops
- EO Noble Camomile: 10 drops
- EO Lemon Eucalyptus: 10 drops

Use: Add 2 drops of this mixture to 2 drops of VO Millerpertuis and massage you around the ear and then drop 1 drop on a cotton swab into the ear canal 3 times a day

GINGIVITIS / canker sore

- EO Tea tree: 10 drops
- EO Laurel: 10 drops

- EO Lavender: 10 drops
- VO Sweet Almond: 20 ml

Use: Apply 2 to 3 drops of this mixture on the affected area and massage gently. Repeat 3 to 4 times per day for 4 days.

STRENGTHENING IMMUNITY (Bath)

- EO Tea tree: 3 drops
- EO Noble Laurel: 3 drops
- EO Ravintsara: 3 drops
- VO Apricot kernel: 10 drops

Use: Mix it in your bath water just before going in.

Ylang Ylang Essential Oil
Scientific name: Cananga odorata
Botanical family: Annonaceae

Stimulating the nervous system, this essential oil is very beneficial against depression and stress. Its exotic and sensual fragrance will enhance your beauty from your skin to your hair.
Main Features:

- Antispasmodic
- Respiratory calming
- Analgesic
- Antidiabetic
- Hair tonic
- Skin tonic
- Tonic, intellectual and sexual stimulant

Therapeutic properties:

Health

- Hypertension, palpitations
- Diabetes
- Spasmodic disorders

Beauty
- Tired skin, dull
- hair loss, dull hair
- Oily scalp

Wellness
- Stress, insomnia
- Sexual asthenia, frigidity

- Depression, anxiety
- Fatigue (physical, nervous and mental)

Precautions: Forbidden in pregnant women, breastfeeding and children under 10 years old. Possible skin irritation for sensitive individuals. Do not intake pure.

Essential oil Ylang Ylang: Recipes

TONING AND SENSUAL BATH

- EO Ylang Ylang: 5 drops
- EO Geranium 2 drops
- EO lavender 1 drop

Use: Add 5 drops of this mix in a tablespoon of vegetable oil in your bath, breathe deeply and relax!

ANGUISH

- EO lavender 1 drop
- EO Ylang Ylang 1 drop
- EO Ravintsara: 1 drop
- VO apricot kernel: 2 drops

Use: Apply 3 drops of the mixture on the solar plexus and the inner wrist, 3 times a day.

TIRED SKIN, TERNE

Use: Add 1 drop of EO Ylang Ylang in your usual cream morning and night.

DISORDERS MENOPAUSE

Use: Add 3 drops of essential oils ylang ylang with vegetable oil and nuts massage the lower abdomen.

DRY HAIR / TERNES

Use: Add 1 drop of EO Ylang Ylang in a usual dose of shampoo, with each washing. Remember to take breaks every 2 to 3 weeks.

HAIR MASK FOR DRY HAIR OR

- EO ylang ylang 30 drops
- EO Laurel: 10 drops
- VO castor: 30 ml
- VO jojoba: 20 ml

Use: Apply the mixture bit by bit on your hair, avoiding the roots. Leave at least 1 hour in a warm towel.

HYPERTENSION, TACHYCARDIA

Use: 1 drop of EO Ylang Ylang on the inside of your wrist and take deep breaths, whenever you feel the need (medical opinion required for use over a long period).

CRISIS OF ANGUISH, STRESS, DEPRESSION, FATIGUE (broadcast)

- EO noble Camomile 3 drops
- EO Lavender 2 drops
- EO Ylang Ylang 2 drops

Use: Pour this mixture into your diffuser to regain calm and energy.

Chapter 3

The best essential oils for your home

As you saw in the previous chapter, essential oils have many properties. If you healing yourself, creating beauty products is possible, why not also use them to take care of your house?

Disinfectant, antiseptic, cleansing, essential oils are used both iasdiffuser, and diluted with other basic household products to maximize their effectiveness or adding up it.

Used in combination with some very economic products such as baking soda or vinegar you can get environmentally friendly household products, economic and highly effective very easily!

Many essential oils can be used as household products, I have, once again, concocted products with our 12 essential oils seen in the previous chapter. Among the essential oils that you can use for your home, we have:

The essential oil of peppermint

Antiseptic; it is very popular to refresh and bring a good scent to your home.

Tip: Spread a few drops of essential oil to get rid of odors after dinner (or a smell of stale smoke!). Its analgesic and toning properties also allow you to relieve your headaches and fight against fatigue!

✿ The essential oil of Tea Tree

Powerful antibacterial, antiviral, fungicide and parasiticide is the multi-use essential oil for your home.

Tip: Mix 10 drops of essential oil to a vegetable oil and put it in your diffuser to sustain a cleaner air in your home.

✿ Essential Oil of Spike Lavender

Antiseptic, Antibacterial, Antiviral and moth, the essential oil of spike lavender is perfectly suited to sanitize and clean your house.

Tip: Mix 8-10 drops of essential oil in hot water after washing your floor clean it is perfect to perfume your home. Its antibacterial and antiviral action will allow you to fight against viral infections in winter!

✿ The essential oil of Ylang Ylang

Relaxing, exotic and delicate fragrance is ideal for scenting your home, your machine and help you be positive by regulating your anxiety!

Tips:

For a perfumed home:
Use pebbles or small pieces of tissue and place a few drops regularly of essential oils to scent your toilet or your closets.

For a scented linen:
In your laundry: add a few drops to your usual detergent
In your iron: Add a few drops in the water in your iron!

Recipes for the maintenance of your home

FLOOR CLEANER

- Washing soda: 2 tablespoons
- Liquid soap 2 tablespoons
- EO noble Laurel: 15 drops
- EO Ylang Ylang 3 drops

> Mix the ingredients in a bucket of warm water before cleaning the floor.

WINDOWS PRODUCT

- White vinegar: 1/3 liter
- Water: 2/3 liter
- EO Eucalyptus 30 drops

> Put the mixture in a 1 liter spray bottle and use it to clean your glass surfaces.

SPRAY MULTI PURPOSE CLEANER

- Sodium bicarbonate: 1 CS
- White vinegar 1 liter
- EO Tea tree: 25 drops
- EO Peppermint: 5 drops

> Mix the ingredients in a spray bottle and apply in areas to clean.

LAUNDRY HOUSE

- Washing soda: 1 glass
- Hot water: 2 cups
- Neutral liquid soap: 1/2 cup
- Baking soda: 1 glass
- EO Tea tree: 8 drops
- EO Ylang Ylang 1 drop

Start by dissolving soda in water then add the liquid soap and baking soda. Add the essential oil of tea tree and ylang ylang and shake to obtain a homogeneous mixture.

> Use a half cup of mixture for each washing machine.

DEODORIZER KITCHEN

EO Lemon Eucalyptus: 25 drops
Vinegar water: 500 ml

> This product can be sprayed on your surfaces, or sprayed in the air to cover the kitchen stubborn odors.

DISHWASHING LIQUID

Baking soda 1 teaspoon
Neutral liquid soap 100 ml
EO of peppermint: 20 drops

> Add the ingredients in a 500 ml pump bottle and fill with water. Shake the bottle before use.

DEODORIZER TOILET

Add 4-5 drops of essential oil of eucalyptus directly into the water after pulling toilet flush to clean and scent your toilet.

DEODORIZER FOR BINS

Mix 5-6 drops of essential oil to 250 ml of warm water and 2 tablespoons neutral liquid soap in a spray bottle. Spray and let dry.

Aromatherapy through the centuries

Aromatherapy is defined by the use of aromatic plant extracts for therapeutic purposes. The word "aromatherapy" comes from the Greek "Aroma" which means "flavor" and "therapeia" comes from the word care, cure. This is one of **naturopathy** resources, unconventional medicine to balance the body by natural means such as diet, lifestyle or herbal medicine (which uses all the elements of a plant). Essential oils can be used for preventive purposes, curative or simply wellness.

The use of plant extracts dates back well before Christ and many civilizations were already using it for many applications.

The use of essential oils Before Christ

More than 4000 years BC, Australian aborigines used it for the treatment of infections. Indians and Chinese had also discovered the therapeutic properties of aromatic essences for millennia.

So this is during the era of ancient Egypt that aromatherapy was developed and used for the first time, in areas as wide as medicine, perfumery, cosmetics or even for embalming the dead. This latter application shows that the Egyptians had already extensive knowledge and anti putrefactive antiseptic essential oils. Their use was very advanced for its time and has influenced many other cultures located on the Mediterranean civilizations such as the Babylonian, Greek and Roman.

300 BC, the essential oils were introduced in Greece by Alexander the Great after his conquest of Egypt. Greek

mythology then attributed these findings to the deities and medicinal plants were then used as an offering to the gods of Mount Olympus. The Romans influenced by the Greeks also used many essential oils particularly in the field of perfumes for men. The virtues of "amorous seduction" of aromatic plants are then known throughout the Roman Empire. In the 1st century after J-C, a doctor, Discoride wrote the book "De Materia Medica", listing more than 520 medicinal plants, which remain the reference to the Renaissance.

In the Middle East, the use of essential oils dates back to 4000 BC, and their use was mainly related to the field of perfumery, until Egyptian influence them do discover other applications especially in medicine . Essential oils were full of magic and their use was first designed to purify the mind before the meeting with the gods, their use was then extended to what we today call "minor injuries."

In the Americas, the uses of essential oils dates back to the Inca civilizations, the Maya and Aztec. Indian tribes still use them today to treat and clean their homes.

From Jesus Christ to nowadays

In the Middle Ages, the essential oils were not used because they were associated with "evil products" and used exclusively by "witches". Herbal remedies were reserved for their monasteries and noble houses. At that time, the research focuses on finding the panacea to become immortal.

Not until the time of the Crusades the interest and the use of essential oils reappeared. The distillation is standard practice and essential oils are then the basis of all remedies through their antibiotic properties that can heal the great epidemics of the time.

Essential oils diffusers are created during the European Renaissance. Called "pomanders" they were used to disinfect houses and people and were widely used to stop the plague.

A well-known story of the time tells the story of four robbers who smeared their body of a brandy particularly anti-infectious, composed of eight essential oils (wormwood, clary sage, rosemary camphor, peppermint, clove, cinnamon, garlic spike and lavender) and then went from house to house, stealing the property of plague victims. During their arrest, they managed to obtain release by offering in exchange the recipe for their potion.

Frantically used by the court of Versailles, including dissemination of powerful odors in the gardens, the French Revolution put an end to the use of fragrances symbol of the French aristocracy. But at the end of the revolution, the bourgeois repossessed perfumes and reused them for themselves.

The birth of scientific aromatherapy

Not until the twentieth century that aromatherapy is recognized as a full medicine. In 1918, a chemist and perfumer named René-Maurice Gattefossé burned his hand during an explosion in his laboratory. He then plunged his hand into a container of essential oil of lavender and finds that the relief is immediate and that healing is excellent. The chemist then devoted himself to studying the antibacterial properties of essential oils. He created in 1928 the word "aromatherapy" followed by a book in which he describes the relationship between the essential biochemical structure of the oil and its business.

In 1929 the pharmacist Sevelinge confirms the high potential antibacterial aromatic substances. Dr. Valnet published in 1964 books that make the public aware of the effectiveness of essential oils. In 1975, Pierre Franchomme highlights the importance of chemotypes that are biologically active molecules in plants. Its precision allows the reduction of failures in therapy as well as reducing the risk of toxicity and side effects.

Aromatherapy then enters the field of science and is part of the natural treatments recognized as the most powerful and effective. Many hospitals use essential oils as disinfectants and also broadcast in some services, to relax patients and cleaner air.

Large plant families in aromatherapy

The vegetable kingdom are over 800,000 species. To classify and identify aromatic plants, botanists use families, genera, species and subspecies. Used both in medicine, in cosmetics and perfumery in gastronomy, herbs are recognized and appreciated worldwide.

If all the plants, flowers, trees and herbs give off an odor, **only 1% of these species can be used to produce essential oils** and are classified into **11 major botanical families.**

Here are the main botanical families of essential oils in this book:

The Lamiaceae or lamiacées (french)

This family includes herbaceous plants or shrubs preferring warm temperated zones and more than 3,500 species distributed in over 200 genres. Plants in this family often have glandular hairs and sub epidermal glands that make them very fragrant, and therefore are very popular in aromatherapy and cosmetics. Grown worldwide, many kinds are present in Europe, notably in the Mediterranean basin.

The main genera of the family Lamiaceae used in aromatherapy are:

✳ **The genus Ocimum**
This genus includes 150 species of herbaceous plants, whose common basil which produces exotic basil EO.

✳ **The genus Lavandula**

This kind brings together the various lavender that produce 3 major essential oils: EO lavender, EO spike lavender and lavender lavendin.

* **The genus Rosmarinus rosemary**

* **The genus Mentha with mints**
This sort has 18 species of mints which 3 are used in aromatherapy:
- Mentha Aquatica: The water mint EO
- Mentha spicata: The EO Peppermint
- Mentha canadensis: The mint EO

* **The genus Origanum Oregano**
Bringing together some fifty species, mostly herbaceous perennials and shrubs, two major species come from this and are widely used both in cooking to flavor dishes that aromatherapy:
- The EO Oregano
- The EO marjoram

* **The genus Salvia with sage**

With over 900 species, sage is appreciated since the Middle Ages for its many medicinal and naturopathic today.The sage EO is extracted from this species.

* **The gender Thymus Thyme**

With over 300 species, thyme is a medicinal plant used since ancient times and known by many civilizations. 4 major essential oils are extracted like this:
- EO Vulgar Thyme thujanol
- EO Thyme satureioide
- EO vulgar Thyme Linalool

- EO vulgar Thyme thymol

Myrtaceae

The myrtle family includes more than 3,000 species of trees and shrubs distributed in a hundred kinds. They are found in temperate, sub-tropical to tropical primarily in Australia, America and Brazil. The species of this family are found in the leaves, flowers, fruit or buds.

In aromatherapy, 4 genera of this family are used for the production of essential oils:

The genus Eucalyptus: Among the 600 species of eucalyptus, only 3 species are used in aromatherapy:
* The Eucalyptus globulus
* The Eucalyptus citriodora
* The Eucalyptus radiata

The genus Melaleuca: 3 species are used for essential oil production:

* The EO Tea tree
* The EO cajeput
* The EO niaouli

The genus Eugenia: Clove essential oil comes from the clove tree native to Indonesia which is also used in gastronomy.

The genus Myrtus: myrtle essential oil is made from a shrub grown for its fruit which are also used in gastronomy and in perfumery.

Asteraceae

This family has the largest number of species with some 13,000 species distributed in 1,500 genera. Present worldwide and in all climates, the distilled part is often found in the flower growing in the grass. Many flowers are Asteraceae (knapweed mountains, dandelion, sunflower or daisy), other vegetables (artichokes, endive) and other medicinal plants.

The essential oils in this family are:

* The noble camomile
* The Immortel

The genus Cinnamomum: Composed of 300 species of trees and shrubs from tropical and warm regions of Southeast Asia, Central America and South America. The essential oils of this type are extracted from the leaves and bark.

* The EO Camphor
* The EO Cinnamon

The Aniba kind which is a species of Amazonian trees and Guyana. So the rosewood EO belongs. This species is threatened, it is best to use essential oil Ho wood.

The kind Laurus nobilis or Laurel is an evergreen shrub species native to the Mediterranean basin. Once used to crown the winners and scientists, where does the name bachelor (bacca laurea: bay laurel). Its leaves are used in cooking (bouquet garni infusion)

Conclusion

Th trend for essential oils is finally a chance for our health and beauty. The media spread the word worldwide highlighting their benefits. Personally I consider this development as a great opportunity. It allows us to emancipate ourselves from the beauty industry and health and its star products, often overpriced and largely inherited from a time when chemistry appeared as the ultimate solution.

The (re) turn to the natural power of plants is likely and that's great !!

Essential oils have many virtues for me. Efficient, versatile, natural, they must find their place in our wellness kit everyday. These advantages, coupled with their limited cost allow each and everyone to afford frequent care, organic and high quality.

During my travels I have often been able to evaluate its power and usefulness. But I also could interact with people from other cultures and the way they use essential oils. This book is the fruit of this mixture: a societal desire to enjoy the benefits of nature, and with the guarantee of a production labeled at a reasonable cost.

All this has produced a practical guide, which has chosen to target the 12 most valuable essential oils! I hope you had as much fun reading it and put it into practice as me to create and to share it with you. If this is the case, then I'm thrilled! You are now "EO" connected !!

If you enjoyed this guide, take a few minutes to leave me a review, it will be a great encouragement to me and will encourage all who seek advice on aromatherapy ... to get started!

www.ingramcontent.com/pod-product-compliance
Lightning Source LLC
Chambersburg PA
CBHW060406190526
45169CB00002B/777